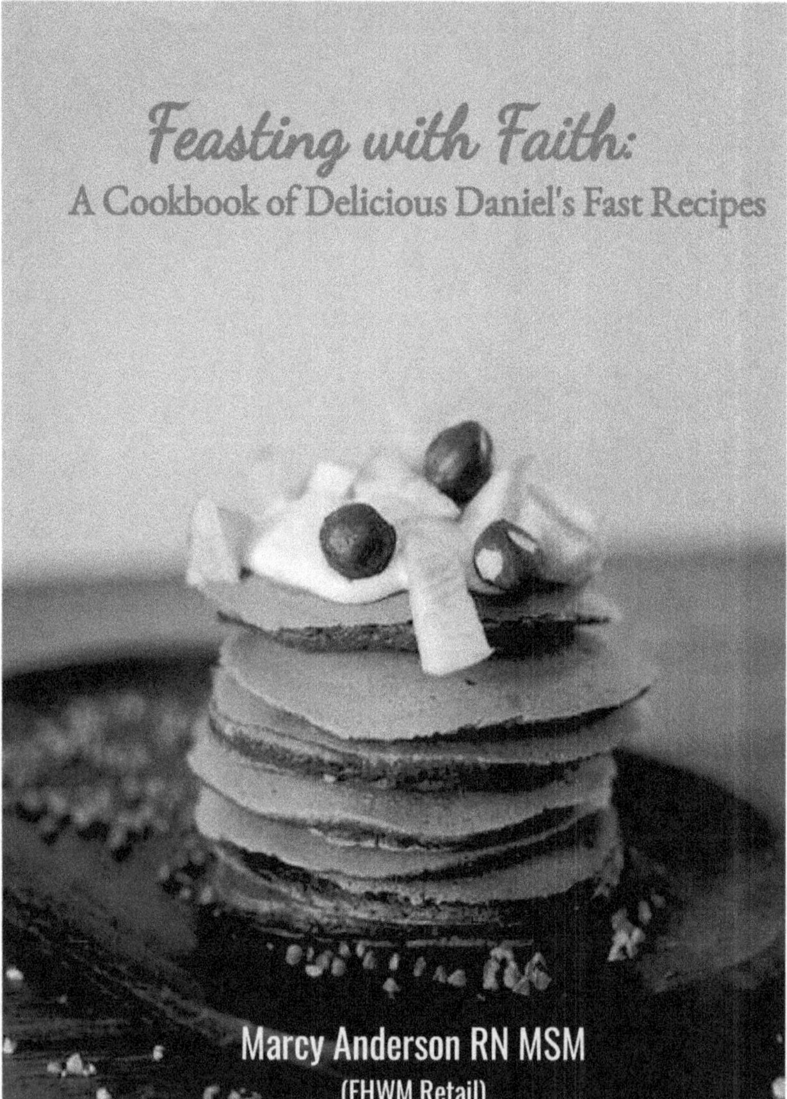


Feasting with Faith:
A Cookbook of Delicious Daniel's Fast Recipes
Marcy Anderson RN MSM
(FHWM Retail)

# Table of Contents




Marcy Anderson RN MSM
(FHWM Retail)

### Introduction:

Are you searching for a cookbook that combines the nourishing benefits of the Daniel's Fast with delicious and healthy recipes? Look no further! We proudly present to you a groundbreaking cookbook authored by a nurse, dedicated to providing you with an exceptional nutrition & culinary experience while prioritizing your health and wellness. Here are compelling reasons why you should add this cookbook, filled with Daniel's Fast healthy recipes, to your collection:

1. Expertise of a Nurse: This cookbook is a culmination of knowledge and experience from a nurse who understands the importance of maintaining a healthy lifestyle. The author's expertise ensures that the recipes are carefully crafted to meet your nutritional needs and support your overall well-being.

2. Daniel's Fast Benefits: The Daniel's Fast is renowned for its ability to cleanse the body and rejuvenate the spirit. By following the Daniel's Fast, you can experience increased energy, improved digestion, weight management, and enhanced mental clarity. This cookbook provides you with a variety of delectable recipes that adhere to the principles of the Daniel's Fast, making it easier for you to embrace this transformative practice.

3. Delicious and Satisfying Recipes: Healthy eating doesn't have to be boring or tasteless! With this cookbook, you'll discover a wide array of mouthwatering recipes that are designed to nourish your body and tantalize your taste buds. From vibrant salads and hearty soups to flavorful main courses and indulgent desserts, each recipe is thoughtfully curated to deliver both nutrition and taste.

4. Easy-to-Follow Instructions: The nurse author understands the demands of a busy lifestyle. That's why this cookbook provides you with easy-to-follow instructions, ensuring that you can effortlessly create delicious meals without spending hours in the kitchen. Whether you're a seasoned chef or a cooking novice, you'll find these recipes accessible and enjoyable to prepare.

5. Varied and Versatile Options: With this cookbook, you'll have an extensive range of recipes at your fingertips. From breakfast options to satisfying dinners and everything in between, you'll never run out of ideas for wholesome and fulfilling meals. The diverse selection of recipes ensures that you can maintain a balanced and exciting diet throughout the Daniel's Fast.

Marcy Anderson RN MSM
(FHWM Retail)

6. Holistic Approach to Health: This cookbook not only focuses on providing nutritious recipes but also emphasizes the importance of holistic well-being.

You'll find helpful tips and insights on mindful eating, self-care practices, and maintaining a positive mindset.

It's a comprehensive guide that nourishes not only your body but also your mind and spirit.

Investing in this cookbook will empower you to embark on a journey towards optimal health and wellness.

By incorporating Daniel's Fast healthy recipes into your daily life, you'll experience the transformative benefits of a balanced diet while enjoying the incredible flavors that nature has to offer. Don't miss out on this opportunity to enhance your culinary repertoire and nourish yourself from within. Order your copy of the Daniel's Fast Healthy Recipes cookbook today and embark on a fulfilling and flavorful adventure towards a healthier you!

**What is the Daniel's Fast?**

In the Bible, the Daniel Fast refers to a specific type of fasting described in the Book of Daniel. The fast is named after Daniel, a prophet and figure in the Hebrew Bible. The guidelines for the Daniel Fast can be found in Daniel 10:2-3:

*"At that time, I, Daniel, mourned for three weeks. I ate no choice food; no meat or wine touched my lips; and I used no lotions at all until the three weeks were over."*

Based on this passage, the Daniel Fast typically involves the following principles:

1. Plant-based diet: The fast emphasizes the consumption of fruits, vegetables, whole grains, legumes, nuts, and seeds. These foods are typically unprocessed and in their natural state.
2. Restriction of animal products: During the fast, followers usually abstain from consuming meat and other animal products such as dairy, eggs, and seafood.
3. Avoidance of processed foods: Processed and refined foods, including added sugars, sweeteners, and artificial ingredients, are typically avoided. The focus is on whole, unprocessed foods.
4. Limited beverages: Some interpretations of the fast also include limitations on beverages, such as avoiding alcoholic beverages and sugary drinks. Instead, individuals may opt for water, herbal teas, or natural fruit juices.
5. It's important to note that interpretations of the Daniel Fast can vary among individuals and religious communities. Some people may adapt the guidelines to suit their specific dietary needs or religious beliefs such as periods of prayer and fasting individually or with a group. If you are considering undertaking the Daniel Fast, it's recommended to consult with a religious leader or trusted authority for guidance and clarification based on your personal needs and religious reliefs.

## Benefits of the Daniel's Fast?

1. Spiritual Discipline: The Daniel Fast can be seen as a spiritual discipline that helps individuals deepen their connection with their faith and cultivate a sense of self-discipline. By committing to the fast, individuals can engage in a period of focused prayer, reflection, and seeking spiritual guidance.  After a fast, many people report a combination of spiritual, physical and mental benefits, including a closer relationship to God, answered prayers, better state of health, freedom from additions, more energy, clearer thinking, feeling lighter and much more!

2. Health Benefits: The Daniel Fast emphasizes the consumption of whole, plant-based foods, which are generally rich in vitamins, minerals, fiber, and antioxidants. By eliminating processed foods, refined sugars, and animal products, the fast promotes a diet that can support weight management, improve heart health, lower cholesterol levels, and enhance overall well-being.

3. Mind-Body Connection: Engaging in the Daniel Fast can foster a greater awareness of the connection between our physical and spiritual well-being. By adopting a healthier dietary pattern, individuals may experience increased energy levels, improved mental clarity, and a heightened sense of vitality. This can positively impact one's ability to engage in spiritual practices and lead a more fulfilling life.

4. Remember, while the Daniel Fast offers potential benefits, it is important to approach any dietary change with consideration for individual health conditions and needs. It's always advisable to consult with a healthcare professional or registered dietitian before starting any new diet or fasting regimen. For example, the types of healthy foods in Daniel's fast such as some nuts may aggravate some conditions such as diverticulosis.

## What Can the Daniel's Fast Provide for You?

1. Guided Meal Planning: A cookbook dedicated to Daniel's Fast diet recipes provides a comprehensive resource for individuals looking to follow this specific dietary approach. It offers a variety of recipes and meal ideas, making it easier to plan and prepare meals throughout the fast. The cookbook can serve as a practical guide, saving time and effort in meal planning.
2. Diverse and Delicious Recipes: The cookbook can introduce individuals to a wide range of flavorful and creative recipes that align with the principles of the Daniel Fast. From breakfast options to main dishes and desserts, the cookbook offers a collection of enticing recipes that cater to different taste preferences, ensuring a satisfying culinary experience throughout the fast.
3. Nutritional Balance and Expertise: A well-designed cookbook dedicated to the Daniel Fast will provide recipes that are carefully crafted to maintain nutritional balance and meet the dietary guidelines of the fast. It can include expert advice, tips, and insights on how to ensure proper nutrition during the fast, making it a valuable resource for those who may be new to this type of dietary practice.
4. Inspiration and Motivation: Having a dedicated cookbook for the Daniel Fast can provide individuals with inspiration and motivation throughout their fasting journey. The visually appealing presentation, personal stories, and testimonials included in the cookbook can encourage individuals to stay committed to the fast, explore new flavors, and embrace a healthier lifestyle.
5. Long-Term Benefits: Even beyond the duration of the fast, the cookbook can serve as a lasting resource for incorporating healthier eating habits into daily life. The recipes and principles of the Daniel Fast can be adapted and integrated into a long-term dietary approach that promotes overall well-being, weight management, and improved health outcomes.

### Other Benefits After Daniel's Fast:
1. Increased Energy
2. Weight Management/Loss
3. Improved Insulin Sensitivity
4. Improved Blood Pressure
5. Mental & Spiritual Clarity

## 10 Daniel's Fast Breakfast Recipes:

1. ***Oatmeal topped with fresh fruits and nuts***: Prepare a bowl of plain oats with water or plant-based milk, and add a variety of chopped fruits like berries, bananas, and apples. Sprinkle some nuts or seeds for added flavor and nutrition.

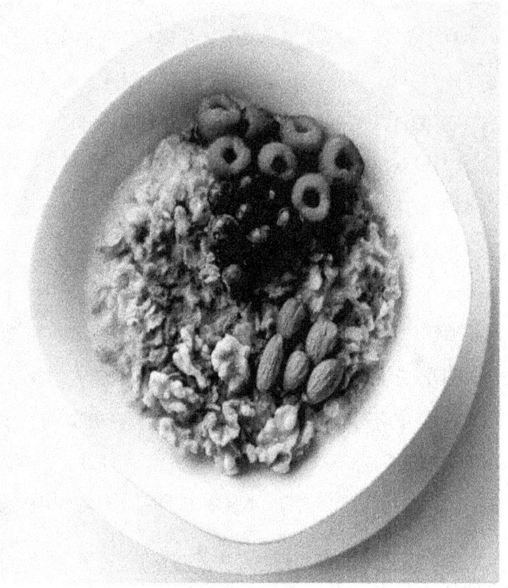

2. ***Whole grain toast with avocado***: Toast a slice of whole grain bread and spread mashed avocado on top. You can also add a sprinkle of salt, pepper, and lemon juice for extra taste.

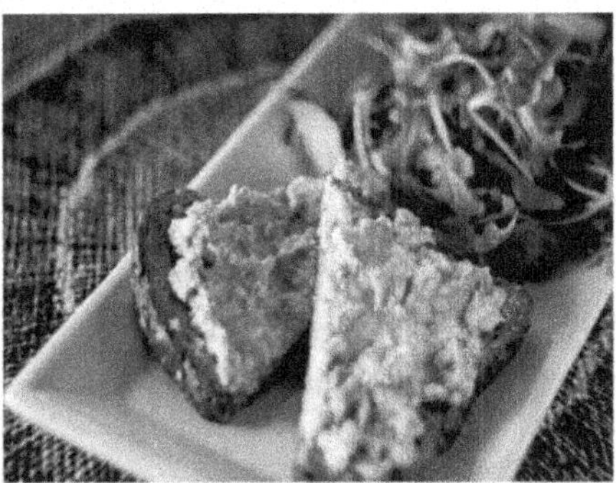

3. ***Fruit smoothie***: Blend together a mix of your favorite fruits such as bananas, berries, mangoes, or pineapples with a liquid base like almond milk or coconut water. You can also add a handful of spinach or kale for added nutrients.

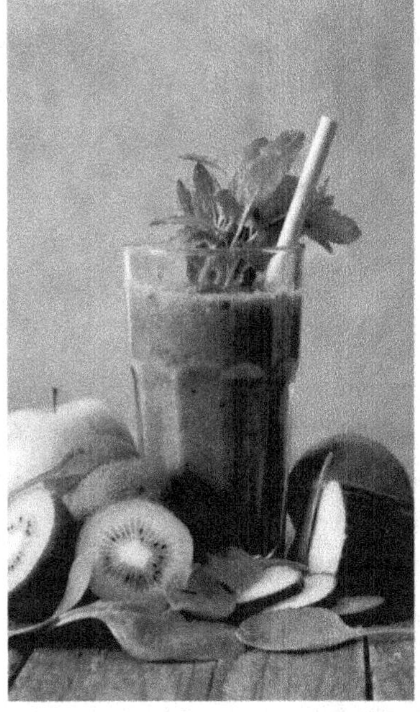

4. ***Chia seed pudding***: Mix chia seeds with plant-based milk (such as almond or coconut milk) and let it sit overnight in the refrigerator. In the morning, top it with fresh fruits, nuts, or shredded coconut.

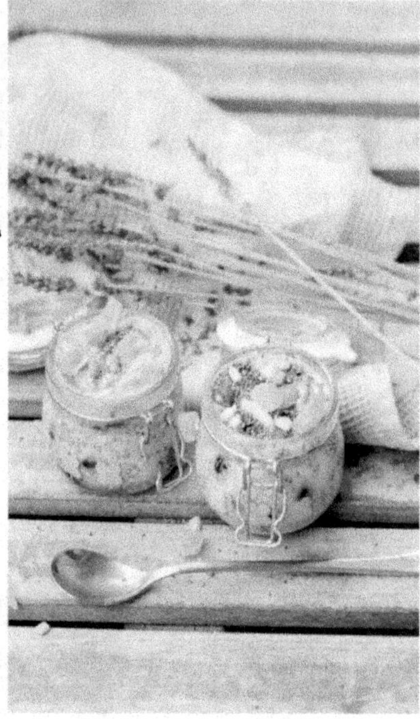

5. ***Vegetable scramble***: Sauté a variety of chopped vegetables like bell peppers, onions, mushrooms, and spinach in olive oil or coconut oil. Season with herbs and spices of your choice, such as garlic, turmeric, and paprika.

6. ***Quinoa breakfast bowl***: Cook quinoa according to package instructions and serve it with a mix of fresh fruits, nuts, and a drizzle of natural sweeteners like maple syrup or honey (if allowed).

7. ***Homemade granola with plant-based yogurt***: Make your own granola using rolled oats, nuts, seeds, and natural sweeteners like honey or dates. Serve it with plant-based yogurt and a side of fresh fruit.

8. ***Buckwheat pancakes***. Prepare pancakes using buckwheat flour, mashed bananas, and plant-based milk. Top them with fresh fruit slices or a small amount of pure maple syrup.

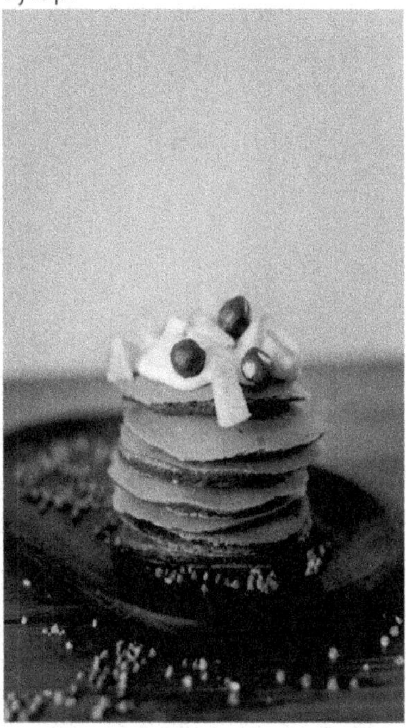

9. ***Veggie wrap***: Fill a whole grain tortilla with a variety of raw or lightly sautéed vegetables, such as cucumber, carrot, bell peppers, and greens. You can also add hummus or mashed avocado for extra flavor.

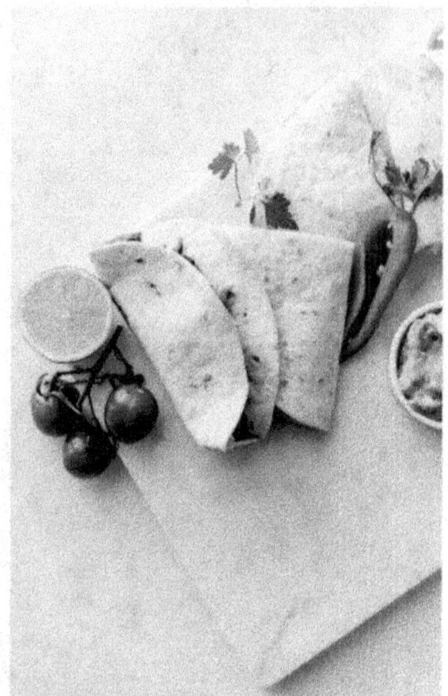

10. ***Overnight oats***: Mix rolled oats with plant-based milk and let it soak overnight in the refrigerator. In the morning, add toppings like sliced fruits, nuts, and a drizzle of natural sweeteners.

**10 Daniel's Fast Lunch Recipes:**

1. *Lentil soup*: Cook a hearty soup with lentils, vegetables like carrots, celery, and onions, and seasonings like garlic, cumin, and turmeric.

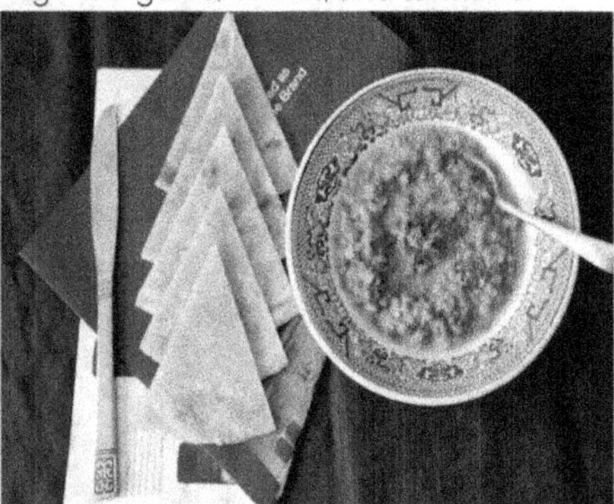

2. *Quinoa salad*: Mix cooked quinoa with chopped vegetables like cucumbers, tomatoes, bell peppers, and herbs like parsley or cilantro. Drizzle with lemon juice and olive oil for dressing.
3. *Baked sweet potatoes with steamed vegetables*: Bake sweet potatoes and serve them with a side of steamed vegetables like broccoli, cauliflower, and carrots.

4. **Chickpea salad**: Combine cooked chickpeas with diced tomatoes, cucumbers, red onions, and fresh herbs. Dress with lemon juice, olive oil, and a pinch of salt.

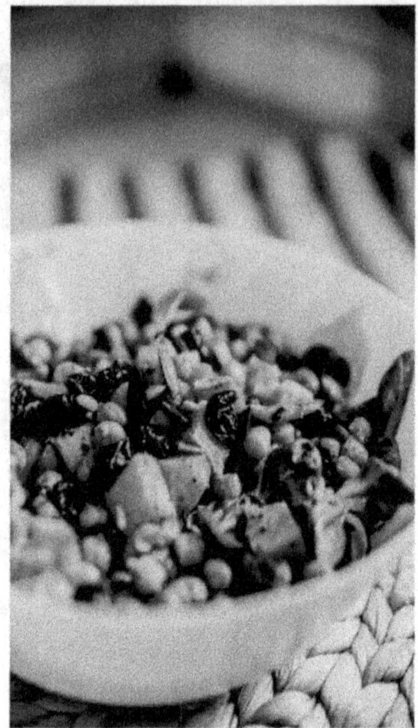

5. **Stuffed bell peppers**: Roast bell peppers and stuff them with a mixture of cooked quinoa, black beans, corn, and diced tomatoes. Bake until tender.

6. ***Mediterranean wrap***. Fill a whole wheat tortilla with hummus, sliced cucumbers, tomatoes, olives, and a sprinkle of feta cheese (if allowed).

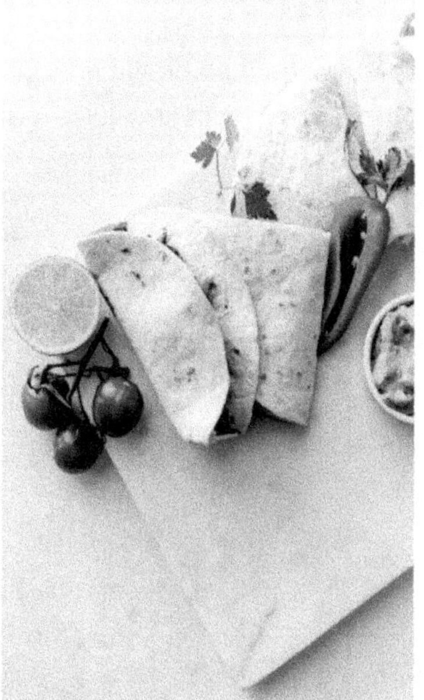

7. ***Vegetable stir-fry***. Sauté a variety of vegetables like broccoli, bell peppers, zucchini, and snap peas in a little olive oil. Add soy sauce or tamari for flavor.

8. ***Lentil salad*** Mix cooked lentils with diced vegetables, such as bell peppers, cherry tomatoes, and red onions. Toss with a vinaigrette made of olive oil, vinegar, and herbs.

9. ***Bean burrito bowl*** Combine cooked brown rice, black beans, corn, diced tomatoes, and avocado. Season with lime juice, cumin, and chili powder.

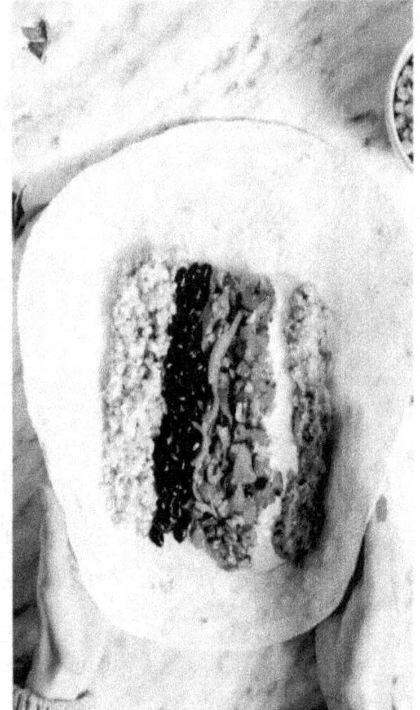

10. ***Grilled vegetable sandwich*** Grill a selection of vegetables like eggplant, zucchini, and bell peppers. Layer them on whole grain bread with hummus or mashed avocado.

## 10 Daniel's Fast Dinner Recipes:

1. ***Baked falafel with quinoa***: Make homemade falafel using chickpeas, herbs, and spices. Serve them with cooked quinoa and a side of mixed greens.
2. ***Ratatouille***: Prepare a traditional ratatouille by stewing a medley of vegetables like eggplant, zucchini, bell peppers, and tomatoes in a flavorful tomato sauce.

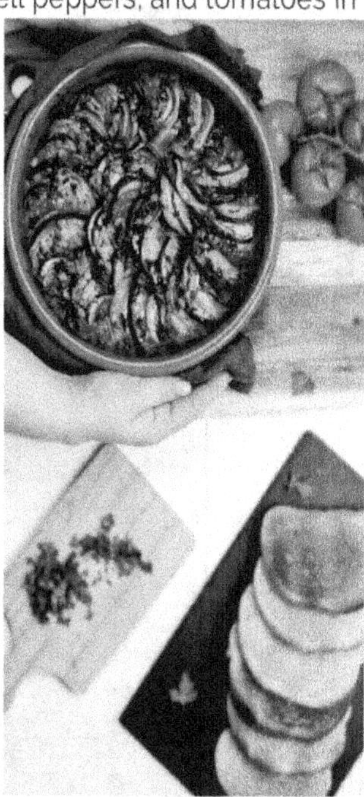

3. ***Spaghetti squash with marinara sauce***: Roast spaghetti squash and use it as a pasta alternative. Top it with a homemade marinara sauce made from fresh tomatoes, garlic, and herbs.

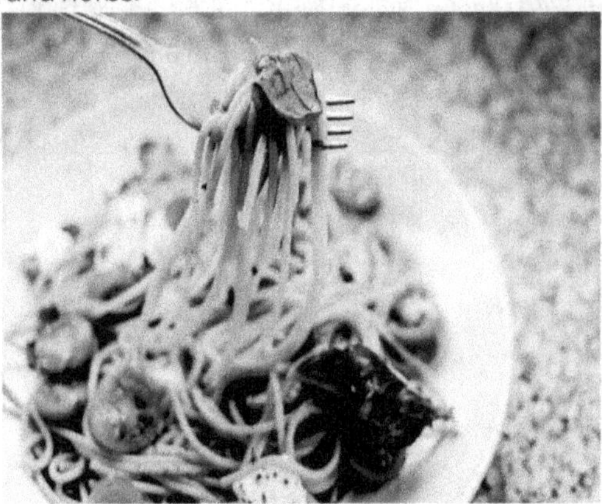

4. ***Stir-fried tofu and vegetables***: Sauté cubed tofu with a variety of vegetables like broccoli, carrots, snow peas, and mushrooms. Flavor it with soy sauce or tamari.

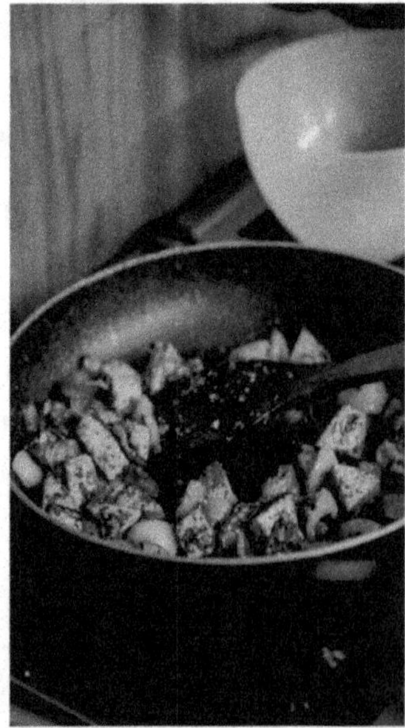

5. ***Stuffed Portobello mushrooms.*** Fill Portobello mushroom caps with a mixture of cooked quinoa, chopped vegetables, and herbs. Bake until tender.

6. ***Veggie curry with brown rice.*** Cook a flavorful vegetable curry using a variety of vegetables like cauliflower, carrots, peas, and bell peppers. Serve it over cooked brown rice.

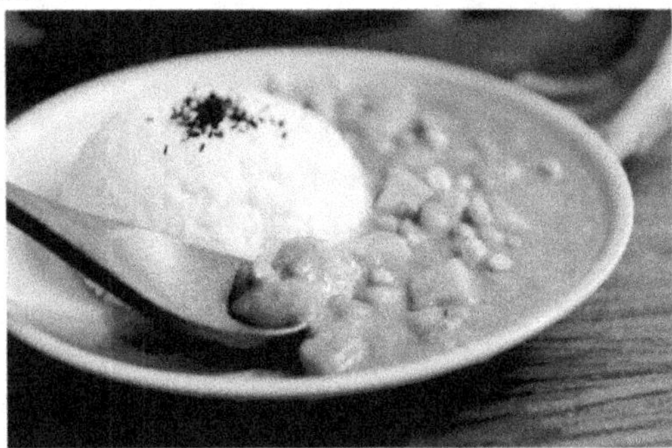

7. ***Lentil and vegetable stew.*** Prepare a hearty stew by combining cooked lentils with a mix of vegetables, such as potatoes, carrots, celery, and onions.

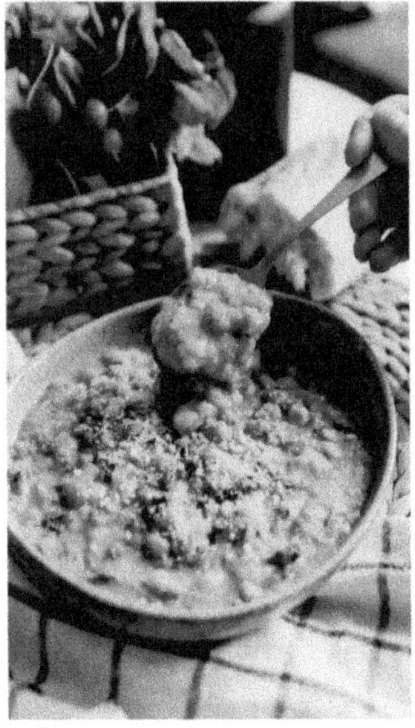

8. ***Baked stuffed bell peppers***. Stuff bell peppers with a filling made from cooked quinoa, black beans, corn, and diced tomatoes. Bake until the peppers are tender.

9. ***Zucchini noodles with pesto***. Spiralize zucchini to create "noodles" and toss them with homemade pesto made from basil, pine nuts, garlic, and olive oil.

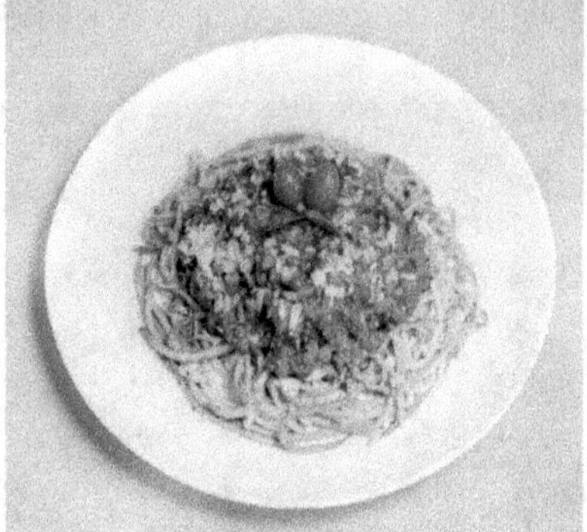

10. ***Grilled vegetable kebabs***. Skewer a variety of vegetables like cherry tomatoes, bell peppers, zucchini, and onions. Grill them until charred and serve with a side of brown rice or quinoa.

**10 Daniel's Fast Desserts:**

You can still enjoy some satisfying and healthy treats that align with the principles of a plant-based diet. Here are ten dessert options that incorporate wholesome ingredients:

1. ***Fruit salad:*** Create a refreshing fruit salad using a variety of seasonal fruits like berries, melons, grapes, and citrus fruits.

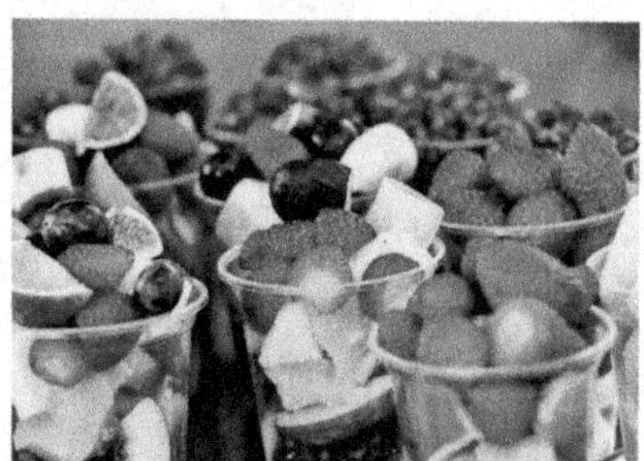

2. ***Baked apples:*** Core and bake apples until tender and sprinkle them with cinnamon and a touch of natural sweetener like honey or maple syrup (if allowed).

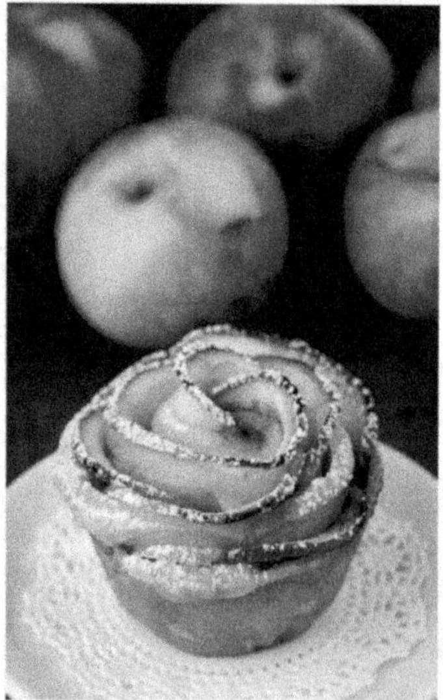

3. **Banana 'nice' cream**: Blend frozen bananas until creamy and smooth to create a dairy-free and naturally sweetened ice cream alternative. Add toppings like nuts, shredded coconut, or cocoa nibs.

4. **Chia seed pudding**: Prepare a delicious chia seed pudding by combining chia seeds with plant-based milk, a natural sweetener, and flavors like vanilla or cocoa powder. Let it set in the refrigerator and top it with fresh fruits.

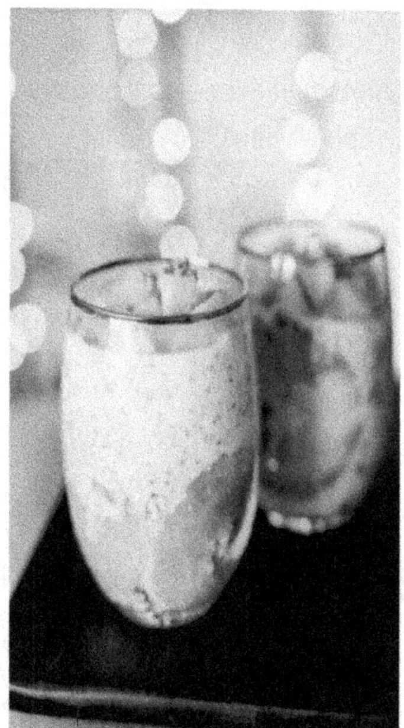

5. **Date energy balls**: Blend dates with nuts, such as almonds or walnuts, and roll them into bite-sized balls. Optionally, you can add cocoa powder or shredded coconut for extra flavor.

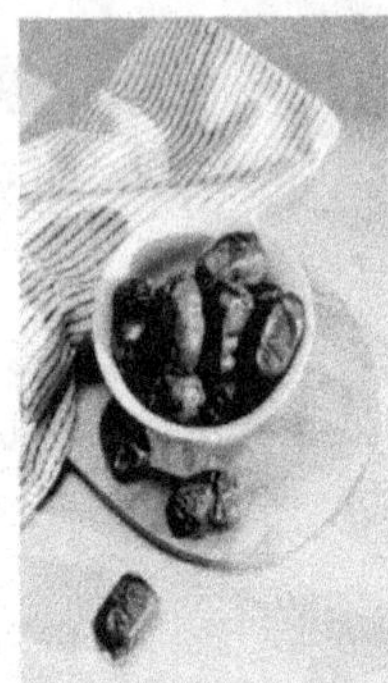

6. ***Baked pears with cinnamon***. Slice pears and bake them until tender. Sprinkle with cinnamon and serve warm.

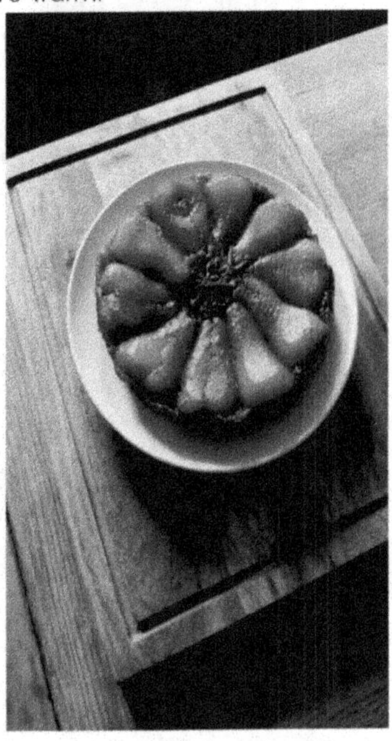

7. ***Mixed berry crisp***. Combine a variety of berries like blueberries, strawberries, and raspberries in a baking dish. Top them with a mixture of oats, almond flour, and a natural sweetener like maple syrup. Bake until golden and bubbly.

8. ***Coconut yogurt parfait***. Layer plant-based yogurt, fresh fruit, and granola in a glass or bowl for a delicious and satisfying dessert option. Adjust fruit choices to your preferences.

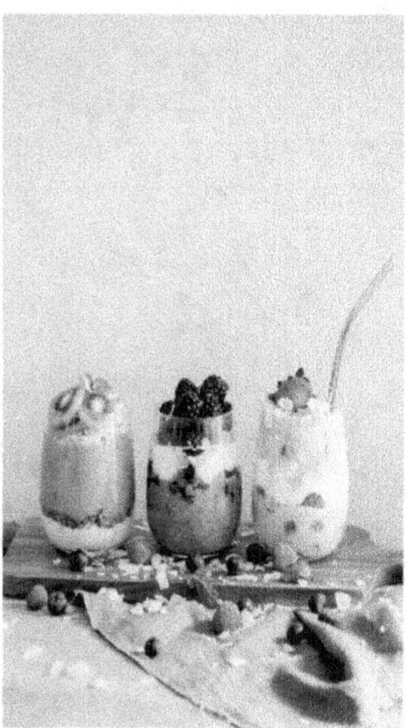

9. ***Almond butter and banana bites***. Slice bananas and spread almond butter between the slices to create little "sandwiches." Optionally, you can dip them in melted dark chocolate and freeze them for a sweet treat.

10. ***Roasted cinnamon chickpeas***. Toss cooked chickpeas with a little oil, cinnamon, and a touch of natural sweetener. Roast them in the oven until crispy for a nutritious and crunchy dessert alternative.

Remember, the Daniel Fast may have variations in interpretation and personal preferences. Adapt these dessert options to suit your specific dietary needs and beliefs.

## 5 Bonus Ideas for Tasty Dishes & Treats:

1. *Sweet Potato and Black Bean Chili:*

- Sauté diced onions, bell peppers, and garlic in olive oil.
- Add diced sweet potatoes, canned black beans (rinsed and drained), diced tomatoes, vegetable broth, and chili powder.
- Simmer until the sweet potatoes are tender and the flavors meld together. Season with salt and pepper to taste.

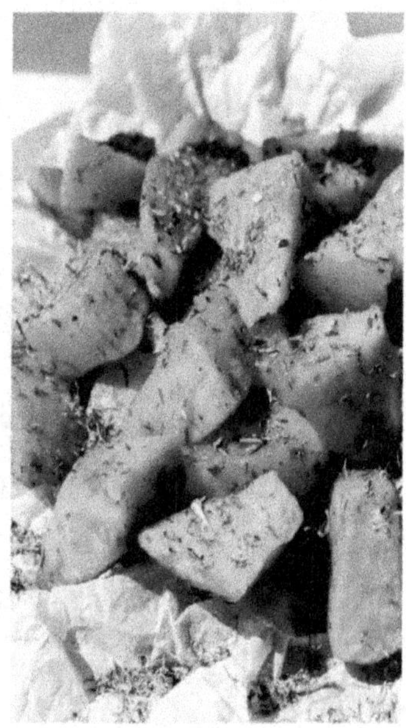

1. *Mediterranean Quinoa Salad.*

- Cook quinoa according to package instructions and let it cool.
- In a large bowl, combine cooked quinoa, diced cucumbers, cherry tomatoes, Kalamata olives, chopped fresh parsley, diced red onions, and crumbled feta cheese (if allowed).
- Drizzle with a dressing made from lemon juice, olive oil, garlic, dried oregano, salt, and pepper. Toss well to combine.

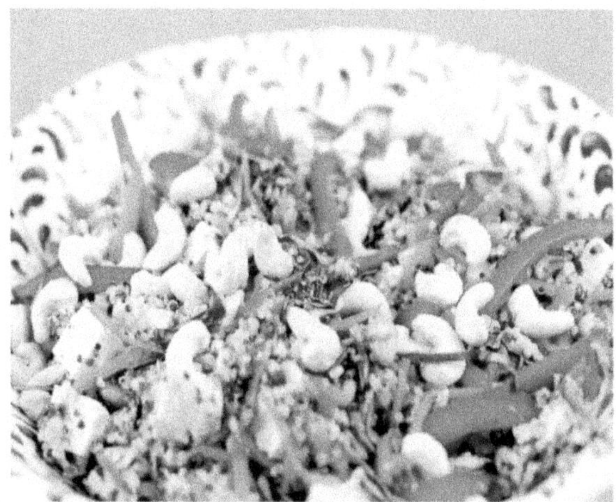

1. *Roasted Vegetable Bowl*

- Toss a selection of chopped vegetables such as sweet potatoes, cauliflower, broccoli, and Brussels sprouts with olive oil, garlic powder, paprika, and salt.
- Spread the vegetables on a baking sheet and roast in the oven until tender and slightly caramelized.
- Serve the roasted vegetables over cooked quinoa or brown rice, and drizzle with tahini dressing.

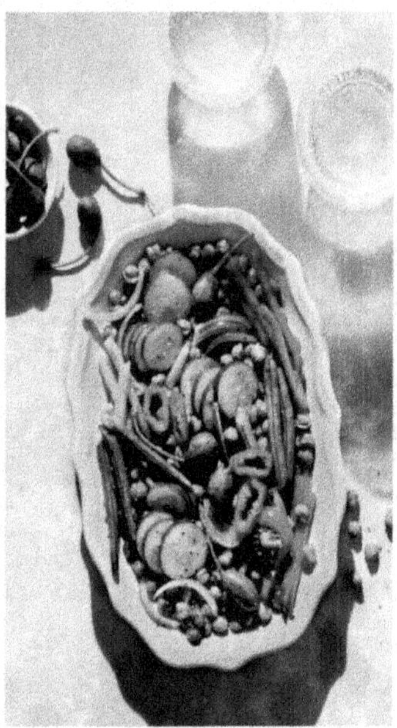

1. *Berry Coconut Chia Pudding.*

- In a jar or container, mix chia seeds with coconut milk, a touch of maple syrup (if allowed), and vanilla extract. Stir well to combine.
- Let the mixture sit in the refrigerator for at least 2 hours or overnight until it thickens.
- Serve the chia pudding layered with fresh berries and a sprinkle of shredded coconut.

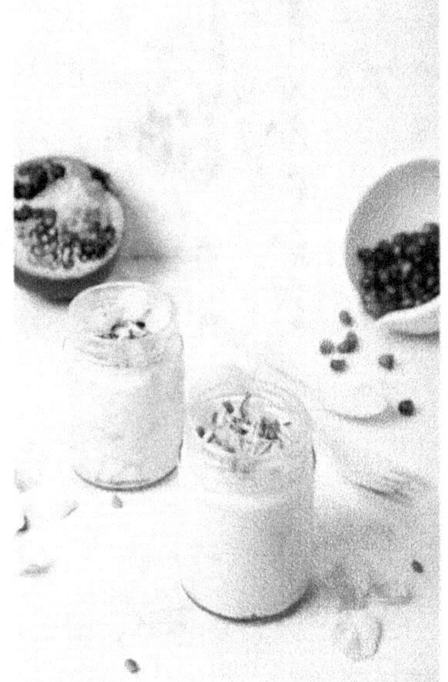

1. *Lentil Curry.*

- Sauté diced onions, garlic, and ginger in a little olive oil until fragrant.
- Add red or green lentils, vegetable broth, diced tomatoes, and a mixture of curry powder, cumin, turmeric, and coriander.
- Simmer until the lentils are cooked and the flavors meld together. Serve over brown rice or quinoa, and garnish with fresh cilantro.

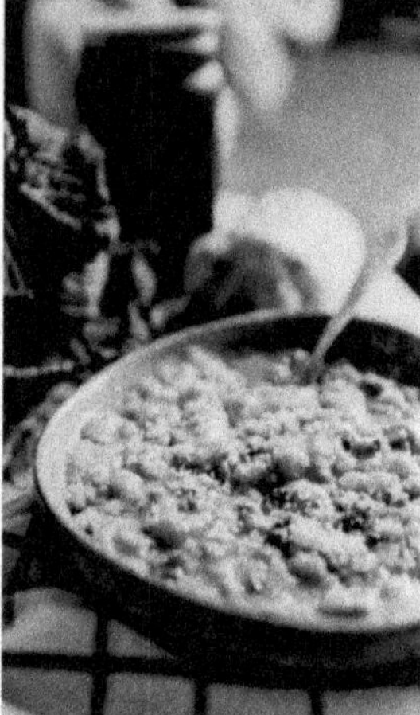

Remember to adjust the recipes according to your personal tastes and dietary needs. Enjoy these flavorful options with your Daniel Fast Recipes!

*The recipe options based on Daniel's Fast principals are unlimited using the guidelines listed at the beginning of the book.

**FHWM Retail LLC** has many platforms designed to support and grow faith, health, wellness & motivation of our consumers, families and communities!

1) First! Check out many of our awesome books, cookbooks, healthcare resources, trackers, journals, diaries & more on Amazon: *https://author.amazon.com/books*. Note; There are also some excellent books found on Send Owl as well: *https://store.sendowl.com/s/df471135-415f-4e0b-9d64-9b159adae6e4*

2) Subscribe to *FHWM with Marcy* on YouTube or *https://youtu.be/EN37UPBcgjA* Our channel is all about fostering holistic wellness through faith, health, and motivation. We believe that taking care of our mind, body, and spirit is crucial for leading a happy and fulfilling life. On our channel, you'll find a variety of content focused on helping you achieve your health and wellness goals. We cover everything from healthy eating and exercise tips to spiritual guidance and motivation. If you're looking to improve your overall well-being and find inspiration and guidance on your journey, then be sure to subscribe to our channel. We can't wait to share our tips and techniques with you and help you become the best version of yourself. Hope to see you as a subscriber soon!

3) Looking for a way to express your faith and connect with like-minded believers? Go to *https://www.fhwmretail.org/* for awesome faith-based merchandise. We offer a wide selection of high-quality products that reflect your love of God and your commitment to living a faithful life. From t-shirts and sweatshirts to active wear and home decor, we have everything you need to show your faith in style. Our products are designed to help you express your faith in a meaningful way, and to inspire others to do the same. Whether you're looking for a gift for a loved one or a treat for yourself, we have something for everyone.

4)  Are you tired of searching for the perfect products to help you achieve your health and wellness goals? Look no further! I am excited to introduce our new online Shopify store!  Go to *https://fhwm-retail.myshopify.com/collections/all* We are dedicated to offering the best products hand-selected by a nurse with over 35 years of experience in the health industry. We understand how important it is to maintain a healthy lifestyle, which is why we have carefully curated a selection of products that are both practical and convenient. Our products are designed to help you incorporate healthy habits into your daily routine without disrupting your busy schedule. One of our featured products is our beautifully crafted alkaline hydrogen water generator. This innovative product allows you to create alkaline hydrogen-rich water, which has been shown to have numerous health benefits, including improving digestion, increasing energy levels, and reducing inflammation. Our store offers many other health convenient products that will help you achieve your wellness goals, from activewear to fitness equipment. We are committed to providing products that are not only effective but also affordable. As a nurse with decades of experience in the health industry, we have seen firsthand the importance of maintaining a healthy lifestyle. Every product in our store has been carefully selected to ensure its effectiveness and practicality.  Thank you for considering our new online Shopify store, and we look forward to helping you achieve optimal health and wellness.

5)  Join us on Twitter: FHWM with Marcy on YouTube @fhwmwithmarcy

- There are more awesome resources coming soon. So, stay tuned!

Holistic Approach to Health: This cookbook not only focuses on providing nutritious recipes but also emphasizes the importance of holistic well-being.  By incorporating Daniel's Fast healthy recipes into your daily life, you'll experience the transformative benefits of a balanced diet while enjoying the incredible flavors that nature has to offer. Don't miss out on this opportunity to enhance your culinary repertoire and nourish yourself from within. Order your copy of the Daniel's Fast Healthy Recipes cookbook today and embark on a fulfilling and flavorful adventure towards a healthier you!